Market Structure as a Determinant of Patient Care Quality

Nathan E. Wilson *†

March 11, 2014

Abstract

Efforts to understand the relationship between market structure and the quality of health services are complicated by the non-random character of patients' choices of where to receive care. To address this problem, I construct an empirical model of health outcomes for dialysis patients that accounts for the endogenous selection of which facility patients choose to receive treatment from. The model's estimates of facilities' average quality are robust to both unobservable variation in condition severity and heterogeneous responses to different facilities' treatment regimes. I estimate the model using data from 2004-2008 for all hemodialysis patients in Atlanta, Georgia. Decompositions of the recovered facility quality estimates show that the average treatment effect is substantially higher in areas characterized by greater competition. Overall, the results suggest that the idiosyncratic match between patient and facility is an important determinant of outcomes, helping to explain the mixed findings in the prior literature.

JEL Codes: C3, I11, L1, L33
Keywords: dialysis, competition, quality, control function, selection bias, random coefficients

---

*The views expressed in this article are those of the author. They do not necessarily represent those of the Federal Trade Commission or any of its Commissioners. Contact: 600 Pennsylvania Avenue NW, M-8059, Washington DC, 20580. Phone: 202-326-3485. E-mail: nwilson@ftc.gov.

†This paper circulated earlier under the title "Market Structure as a Determinant of Patient Care Quality: Evidence from the Retail Dialysis Sector." I am extremely grateful for help and comments from many of my colleagues as well as Lapo Filustrucchi, Paul Grieco, Nathan Miller, Chris Ody and commenters at the University of Michigan, University of New Mexico, and 2013 International Industrial Organization Conference. The usual caveat applies.

1 Introduction

Today, nearly 400,000 Americans regularly receive dialysis to compensate for having permanently lost kidney function. The cost of such care averages almost $80,000 per person per year, most of which is paid for by Medicare. As a result, spending on End Stage Renal Disease (ESRD) accounted for close to 1% of the entire Federal budget in 2010 (Ramanarayanan and Snyder, 2012). Despite efforts by the Centers of Medicare and Medicaid to ensure a high return on these expenditures, commentators have complained for decades that the average quality of hemodialysis treatment in America lags that of other developed nations while also exhibiting considerable variation from facility to facility (Relman and Rennie, 1980, Fields, 2010a,b). These concerns have given rise to a large scholarly literature aimed at uncovering the determinants of quality in the industry.

Notwithstanding the attention, little is well-accepted about whether or not dialysis patients' outcomes vary with factors like the degree of local competition. At first, the marked lack of consensus may seem surprising. After all, most economic models strongly predict that quality should be positively related to competition when prices are administratively determined (Gaynor, 2006).[1] However, given the reasonable expectation that patients select to receive treatment from the facilities most likely to benefit them, it is difficult for analysts to believe that comparing facilities' average outcomes will reveal the causal impact of different facility or market characteristics.[2] For example, if more competitive markets leads to higher service quality, and unobservably sicker patients systematically prefer higher quality, then simple analyses of the impact of market structure on average quality will be biased.

Concern about bias due to patients' unobserved condition severity is longstanding in the health economics literature. However, one might also worry about selection due to differences in how individuals respond to different providers. For example, one factor affecting health outcomes might be how well patients follow their clinicians' instructions, which could

---

[1]Katz (2013) notes that under certain circumstances this relationship may fall apart, but that increases in concentration as a result of acquisitions are invariably associated with lower incentives to provide high quality care.

[2] See, e.g., Romano and Mutter (2004) on the merits of various quality metrics.

be unobservably influenced by demographic similarities between patients and providers. If patients take this into account, it could produce idiosyncratic patient-facility matching that could also lead to biased estimates of the relationship between competition and average treatment quality if multi-facility firms specialize in different types of patient and collocate facilities close to a group of them.

Even though dialysis is often thought of as an undifferentiated service, the medical literature has documented significant heterogeneity in centers' styles of treatment as well as patients' responses to those different treatment regimes. Thus, there are grounds for expecting patient-facility matching to be an economically important determinant of outcomes. Despite this, the past literature on dialysis quality has never sought to control for it. To address the gap and estimate the relationship between market structure and treatment quality, while accounting for both patients' unobserved condition severity and the possibility of heterogeneous treatment response, I develop a multi-stage empirical model. It provides unbiased estimates of facilities' average quality to be decomposed upon market structure proxies. The precise steps in the model are as follows.

First, I exploit detailed patient-level data on the facility choices and health outcomes of all ESRD patients receiving hemodialysis treatment in the metro Atlanta area between 2004 and 2008. After cleaning, there are almost 25,000 patient-year observations associated with just under 100 different facilities. These highly detailed data permit me to explicitly model the facility selection process as in the hospital choice literature (Capps et al., 2003, Ho, 2006).

Second, I develop a control function (CF) approach to estimate the average quality of many different endogenous treatments that draws on the facility choice results to infer information about patients' unobservable characteristics. The CF estimator integrates insights from previous papers in the labor and marketing literatures where one or two endogenous variables are allowed to have heterogenous coefficients with past work on Roy models that accomodate the possibility of a multinomial selection problem.[3] The key to the estimator is

---

[3]Key past and recent papers on heterogeneous treatment effects include Heckman (1978), Card (2001), Luan and Sudhir (2010), Petrin and Train (2010), while relevant multinomial Roy model papers include Lee

its exploitation of the well-known stylized fact that patients prefer to receive treatment close to their homes to infer that patients who choose to receive treatment at distant facilities likely have unobservable expectations of better outcomes there.[4]

Third, I collect the estimated facility-specific effects from the outcome model, which constitute a selection-corrected quality index, and decompose them on facility- and market-level factors to identify any relationship between quality and market or organizational structure. This approach is similar to that used in the structural productivity literature (Syverson, 2011), and a somewhat similar tactic was previously employed to analyze hospital quality by Gowrisankaran and Town (1999). Decomposing the CF estimates addresses the chief problem associated with market structure regressions, which is that structure reflects unobserved differences in the outcome variable. Since the quality metric produced by the CF model explicitly accounts for the endogenous composition of the patient population seen at a given facility, one need not worry about this form of endogeneity. In effect, the model conditions out the possibility that facilities collocate with patients who will disproportionately benefit from treatment at them.

My analysis of the Atlanta data strongly suggests, first, that patients do heterogeneously respond to treatment at different facilities. In other words, different patients with the same underlying level of condition severity would expect to consistently have different outcomes from frequenting the same facility. Evidence for this can be seen in the fact that formal and informal specification tests support the usage of the CF specification relative to simpler, but potentially more efficient models. Moreover, a direct test of the behavioral assumption underpinning the CF model does not reject it.

Second, my decomposition results imply that competition is both an economically and statistically significant determinant of average treatment quality. For example, my baseline estimates imply that if a multi-center firm acquires one additional existing facility in the average market that it would increase the expected number of days that the average patient

---

(1978, 1983), Dahl (2002), Beaudry et al. (2007, 2010).

[4]Gowrisankaran and Town (1999), Kessler and McClellan (2000), Gaynor et al. (2005), Brooks et al. (2006), Ho (2006), Lee et al. (2010).

4

would spend in the ICU or CCU by 28% and increase the probability of death by 7 percentage points. Finally, I find no statistically significant evidence that for-profit status is associated with a different level of average treatment quality.

Interestingly, when I decompose quality estimates that control for variation in patient condition severity, but not idiosyncratic patient-facility matching, I find much that concentration has a much smaller impact on quality. For example, the results predict that a facility acquisition in the mean market would only increase the expected number of days spent in the ICU or CCU by 3%. The smaller impact of a change in competition on the quality of treatment on the treated (after adjusting for selection based on unobservable differences in condition severity) is consistent with multiproduct firms diversifying their product space to appeal to heterogeneous consumers (see, e.g., Salop (1979), Shaked and Sutton (1982)). Moreover, it helps to explain why the dramatic increase in concentration that the industry has undergone in recent years has not produced the dramatically worse outcomes implied by the baseline estimates.

My results about the relation between market structure and treatment quality differ significantly from many of those in the prior literature, which have tended to find no statistically significant relation between competition and quality while often suggesting that for-profit centers provide worse service (Grieco and McDevitt, 2012, Cutler et al., 2012, Garg et al., 1999, Devereaux et al., 2002, Zhang et al., 2011).[5] By varying my empirical specifications, I am able to largely explain the apparent discrepancy. For example, the previous findings stem from empirical strategies or datasets that do not accomodate accounting for the importance of unobserved patient characteristics and their idiosyncratic match with different facilities. When I use such "raw" quality estimates, I also find no significant relationship between concentration and quality, which is consistent with the hypothesis that sicker patients seek out higher quality facilities, downwardly biasing the estimated impact of competition on quality.

Overall, the paper contributes to the growing literature using alternatives to the stan-

---

[5]I should note that Brooks et al. (2006) also found that for-profit centers do not consistently provide worse quality after addressing the possibility of unobserved variation in condition severity with a distance-based IV strategy.

dard instrumental variables (IV) framework to address endogeneity concerns (Dustmann and Meghir, 2005, Liu et al., 2010, Luan and Sudhir, 2010). It extends the existing approaches to accomodate the possibility of polychotomous treatments, an important issue in health care and industrial organization. In addition, the paper adds to the rapidly expanding literature on the importance of market structure in health care settings (Gaynor and Town, 2011), focusing on a comparatively understudied industry relative to its impact on patient lives and the Federal budget. In the dialysis setting, the paper's results appear to validate the concern of antitrust regulators about the consequences of increasing concentration in narrowly defined geographic markets and reconcile why the prior literature had not found the theoretically predicted result.[6]

The remainder of the paper is organized as follows. Section 2 describes the institutional setting of the dialysis industry, paying special attention to the prior evidence of heterogeneous treatment effects. Section 3 presents the empirical model, discussing identification and the relationship to the prior literature. Section 4 describes the data. Section 5 presents the results of the treatment outcome models, focusing on the evidence for inferring the existence of idiosyncratic matching between facilities and patients. Section 6 shows the results of decompositions of facilities' quality on measures of market structure. Section 7 concludes.

2 Background

2.1 Industry Characteristics

A diagnosis of ESRD means that an individual has permanently lost kidney function.[7] ESRD generally arises as a consequence of chronic kidney disease, coronary disease, hypertension, diabetes, and other progressive, chronic conditions. The incidence – meaning the commonality of new diagnoses – of ESRD has risen dramatically. Between 1980 and 2008, just the

---

[6] For example, the Federal Trade Commission (FTC) recently required that DaVita sell off 29 dialysis centers in order to preserve competition in 22 different local markets. See http://www.ftc.gov/opa/2011/09/davita.shtm.

[7] For in depth treatments of ESRD, see Farley (1993), Wilson (2013), or the citations therein.

newly diagnosed sufferers' share of the total U.S. population increased from less than 0.1 percent to 0.35 percent (USRDS, 2011). This dramatic increase has had grave implications for Federal expenditures, because all Americans suffering from ESRD are eligible to receive Medicare benefits without regard to age or other factors.[8]

Invariably fatal without treatment, ESRD can be treated either through chronic dialyzation or transplant. Given the marked lack of kidneys available for transplant, the vast majority of ESRD patients regularly receive some form of dialysis. By far the most common dialysis modality ($\approx 90\%$ of patients) is hemodialysis, which pumps patients' blood through a machine that replicates the cleaning process typically performed by functioning kidneys. Though sometimes done in hospitals, patients generally undergo hemodialysis treatment in specialized facilities supervised by clinicians.[9] These facilities are not terribly large in size, as can be seen in Figure 1, and tend either to be stand-alone buildings or to occupy a portion of a strip mall. As for other industries, Medicare sets the price for hemodialysis services administratively, allowing industry analysts to focus on quality in isolation from pricing.[10]

Although the industry was initially fairly atomistic (Farley, 1993), by the 21st century, the market to provide hemodialysis services had become extremely concentrated (Wilson, 2013). For example, the two leading for-profit chains' share of facilities reached almost 60 percent by the end of 2008. The two firms' growth has been achieved through a combination of "organic" growth via the opening of new facilities, and by acquiring other for-profit chains via a series of mergers (Pozniak et al., 2010, Cutler et al., 2012). Unsurprisingly, many of the more recent mergers have drawn scrutiny from antitrust enforcement agencies.

Overall, the massive consolidation of the industry suggests that controlling for the possibility of different impacts from the proximity of facilities under different types of ownership is a potentially important element in understanding the impact of market structure on treat-

---

[8]Medicare covers approximately 80 percent of treatment costs; patients cover the remainder out of pocket, or through supplemental insurance policies. For in-clinic dialysis, Medicare covers exactly 80 percent. For additional copay information, see, e.g., http://www.carepathways.com/MedicareCoverage.cfm.

[9]The most common alternative modality is peritoneal dialysis, wherein patients receive injections of a cleansing dialysate that must be replaced every few hours. This may occur either in patients' homes or in facilities. For more details on treatment modalities, see http://www.usrds.org/2012/view/v2_01.aspx.

[10]For lengthier discussion of payment details, see Wilson (2013) and citations therein. For an analysis of the impact of dialysis provider concentration on private insurers, see Cutler et al. (2012).

ment quality.

2.2 Dialysis Treatment Heterogeneity and Sorting

Though dialysis is often thought of as a fairly undifferentiated service, many medical researchers have documented substantial heterogeneity in how it is provided and how patients respond.

First, some studies have shown heterogeneous response to broadly equivalent treatment. For example, Henderson (1986) found that different ESRD patients receiving the same type of hemodialysis nevertheless had quite distinct outcomes when given hemofiltration treatments, and that these outcomes could not be strongly correlated with the hypothesized covariates. The study suggests that seemingly similar dialysis patients may be quite different, and may respond in heterogeneous manners to even standard treatments. Focusing on peritoneal dialysis, a type of dialysis modality more popular in other parts of the world, Kagari et al. (1993) also find wide variation in peritoneal dialysis patients' outcomes. They conclude that "inherent constitutional factors may be responsible for some of the observed heterogeneity" [p .32] . Consistent with this view, Schaefer et al. (1991) found that techniques for classifying patients based on observable characteristics did too poor job of predicting the needs of ESRD patients admitted to an ICU to be used to guide clinical decision-making.

Second, a number of papers have surveyed patients' responses to different styles of dialysis treatment. Many of the early contributions in this vein were surveyed in Jones (1992), who notes considerable variation across facilities in the costliness of their treatment programs as well as other characteristics of their treatment regimes. While Jones (1992) did not find that such differences led to consistent differences in outcome, many subsequent papers have identifiied such findings, exploiting apparently wide variation in common practice. For example, Phrommintikul et al. (2007) conduct a meta analysis of studies of the impact of a key pharmaceutical hemodialysis treatment on different types of patients, and conclude that a naive prescription of similar doses across patients would have adverse outcomes for some patient types. Similarly, Schiffl et al. (2002) used a meta-analysis to conclude that patients suffering acute renal failure benefited from more regular treatment.

Given such heterogeneity in outcomes and treatment styles, it is perhaps unsurprising that researchers have also documented evidence of non-random matching between patients and facilities. For example, Zhang et al. (2011) finds that the hypothesis that different for-profit chains' patient populations are equivalent is rejected at the 1% level across a wide variety of demographic factors. Such sorting behavior might reflect some facilities efforts to specialize in treating certain types of patients

Overall, while not constituting direct evidence of variation in treatment effects across facilities, the prior literature does provide strong circumstantial grounds for believing that heterogeneous treatment effects may be of economic significance in understanding outcomes and behavior in this industry. Below, I describe how one might account for this possibility when empirically estimating the average quality of treatment.

3 The Empirical Model

Consistent with the prior literature on patients' choices (see, e.g., Gowrisankaran and Town (1999), Kessler and McClellan (2000), Geweke et al. (2003)), I assume the effects of dialysis facility selection on health outcomes can be modeled in discrete time, and that each period's decisions are independent of those that come before. Within a period, a multi-stage game maps from facilities' and patients' choices to patient outcomes.

3.1 Facility Selection & Treatment Outcome

For expositional purposes, I begin with a simplified setting with just two possible places to receive treatment: A and B. The goal of estimation is to identify the quality of A relative to B. In describing how this inference might be drawn, I broadly follow the expositional approach taken in previous papers concerned with stochastic treatment effects (Card, 2001, Luan and Sudhir, 2010).

Within a given period, the game proceeds as follows. In the first stage, facilities determine what type of treatment they wish to provide, choosing a single quality type, which may heterogeneously impact patients. In practical terms, this may be thought of as developing expertise in certain types of patients. Once their choice has been made, facilities are not able to customize their quality to each patient's characteristics.

In the second stage, an individual requiring dialyzation decides which facility they will visit for treatment after having observed facilities' quality decisions. Once the choice of facility is made, the treatment outcome y_i is realized for patient i.

Defining c_i to be an indicator variable taking the value of one if patient i receives treatment at facility A, one can obtain the relative benefit of receiving treatment at A by estimating the following treatment equation:

$$y_i = f(c_i, x_i | \theta_i) + \epsilon_i, \tag{1}$$

where x_i are observable confounding factors, θ_i is a vector of parameters possibly unique to patient i, $f(\cdot)$ is a possibly nonlinear function of the inputs, and ϵ is information unobservable to the econometrician.

If one makes the standard assumption that the inputs to $f(\cdot)$ enter linearly, Equation (1) can be rewritten as:

$$y_i = f(\theta_{i1} + \theta_{i2}c_i + x_i\theta_3) + \epsilon_i,$$

where the lack of a patient-specific subscript on θ_3 indicates that it is constant across the population. Following Card (2001), the elements of this equation can be divided to separate the individual-level heterogeneity from the mean effects of the different regressors:

$$y_i = f(\theta_{01} + \bar{\theta}_2 c_i + x_i\theta_3 + \tilde{\theta}_{i1} + (\theta_{i2} - \bar{\theta}_2)c_i) + \epsilon_i, \tag{2}$$

where $\tilde{\theta}_{i1} = \theta_{i1} - \theta_{01}$ and has mean 0.

Now, assume (as in Berry et al. (1995)) that the heterogeneity in the coefficients can be parameterized as linear functions of the observable factors x_i and some unobservable, stochastic elements.[11] This means that the random coefficients in Equation (2) can be rewritten as:

$$\tilde{\theta}_{i1} = x_i \beta^1 + \phi_i^1, \text{ and} \tag{3}$$

$$(\theta_{i2} - \bar{\theta}_2) = x_i \beta^2 + \phi_i^2. \tag{4}$$

In this case, β^1 indicates how the observable factors relate to variation in expected outcomes at the patient-level, while β^2 reflects how the observables alter the marginal effect of receiving treatment at facility A. The ϕ capture the influence of unobservable information on patients' heterogeneity, both in terms of underlying condition severity and responsiveness to treatment at A.

So long as the choice of treating facility is exogenously determined, the assumption that the θ_i are linear functions implies that Equation (2) can be consistently estimated via ordinary least squares (OLS) if $f(\cdot)$ is a linear function.[12] However, problems arise if the choice of treatment facility is non-random. The most natural way of understanding this in the dialysis context would be if the patient – or their referring nephrologist – possesses insight into the unobserved information (i.e., θ_{i1}, θ_{i2}, or ϵ_i) in the treatment equation. Knowledge about these parameters would then be expected to affect the choice of facility. If the goal is to subsequently evaluate what factors may be influencing $\bar{\theta}_2$, such bias is of major concern.

There is a large literature in health care suggesting that this sort of selection bias occurs and has economically meaningful effects on estimates if left unaddressed (Gowrisankaran and Town, 1999, Kessler and McClellan, 2000, Geweke et al., 2003, Varkevisser et al., 2012). To address the problem, health economists have typically turned to IV methods, which allow the endogenous choice of treating facility to be correlated with the random intercept term θ_{i1} in Equation (2). In other words, these approaches control for the possiblity of unobserved variation in condition severity, but preclude the possibility of heterogeneous treatment effects (i.e., $\theta_{i2} \neq \bar{\theta}_2$).

---

[11]In practice, it is likely that only a subset of the observables x impacts the random coefficients; however, for notational ease, I simply use x.

[12]If f is nonlinear, however, it may still be estimated consistently using standard simulation approaches to dealing with random coefficients in nonlinear models (see, e.g., Train (2003)).

Thus, the standard approach to dealing with individual-level unobserved heterogeneity addresses the concern that sicker patients will choose better facilities (i.e., *intercept endogeneity*), but leaves unaddressed any problems stemming from variation in responsiveness to facilities' treatments (i.e., *slope endogeneity*) (Luan and Sudhir, 2010). Worrisomely, this means that not only will estimation methods that ignore any possibility of selection bias give inconsistent estimates of the average treatment effect, but so too will the standard IV estimator (Card, 2001).[13] Instead of providing insight into the average treatment effect, IV estimation will instead give an estimate of the average effect of treatment on the treated after (at least partially) adjusting for unobserved condition severity. To be sure, this is of interest, especially since patients and their nephrologists often play an active role in selecting their treatment location. However, it is distinct from the question of how competition affects average treatment quality.

I address the problem of accurately inferring average treatment quality by using an approach that permits both random parameters, θ_{i1} and θ_{i2}, to influence the choice of treatment facility c_i. I begin – as in standard IV – by assuming that the choice of facility, c_i, is a function not just of the observables included in Equation (1), but also a set of exogenous variables z_i that do not influence y_i except through their influence on c_i (i.e., instruments). Health scholars have long assumed that patients' travel distances satisfy these criteria, as the selection of a treating facility will be influenced by the patient's travel cost of reaching it, but travel distance should not independently influence their outcomes.[14] Thus, using a linear probability model, the likelihood that a patient elects treatment at A can be written as:

$$c_i = z_i\gamma + \eta_i. \tag{5}$$

Provided that the choice model is correctly specified, the error term should be uncorrelated with the instruments, i.e., $E[\eta|z] = 0$.

---

[13]Moreover, even if there is no slope endogeneity (i.e., $\beta_{i2} = \bar{\beta}_2 \forall i$), standard IV estimation will lead to inconsistent estimates if f is nonlinear as shown in Terza et al. (2008a,b).

[14]See, e.g., Gowrisankaran and Town (1999), Kessler and McClellan (2000), Gaynor et al. (2005), Brooks et al. (2006), Ho (2006), Lee et al. (2010).

One additional assumption is required before the treatment equation can be estimated. This critical requirement is that the unobservables from Equations (3) and (4) are mean independent of the instruments z_i after conditioning on η_i. Formally, this means that $E[\phi|z, \eta] = E[\phi|\eta]$. In practice, the identifying assumption underlying this model is that the stochastic heterogeneity in responsiveness to treatment, ϕ^2, can be modeled as a function of the random elements impacting the choice of facility, η, and that distance itself does not impact treatment responsiveness. In other words, $E[\phi|\eta] = g(\eta)$. In the context of dialysis facility choices, these assumption add up to a very intuitive story: if a patient's observables suggest that she should choose treatment at facility A, but she does not, then this likely reflects something correlated with her expected outcome from treatment there. She must expect to receive better treatment elsewhere or else it would not be worth incurring higher costs to go there. This logic is very similar to that used to endogenize work location when considering the impact of different factors on wages (Dahl, 2002, Beaudry et al., 2007, 2010).

Altogether, these assumptions, and the convention of assuming that the conditional expectation can be modeled using its linear approximation (Petrin and Train, 2010), imply that Equations 3 and 4 can be rewritten as:

$$\tilde{\theta}_{i1} = x_i\beta^1 + \phi_i^1 = x_i\beta^1 + \psi\eta_i, \text{ and} \tag{6}$$

$$(\theta_{i2} - \bar{\theta}_2) = x_i\beta^2 + \phi_i^2 = x_i\beta^2 + \tau\eta_i. \tag{7}$$

To empirically implement the estimator, one replaces the ηs in Equations (6) and (7) with the unbiased estimates produced by estimating Equation (5). Thus, the CF treatment equation becomes:

$$y_i = f(\theta_{01} + \bar{\theta}_2 c_i + \overbrace{\psi\hat{\eta}_i + \tau\hat{\eta}_i c_i}^{\text{control function}} + x_i\tilde{\theta}_3) + \epsilon_i, \tag{8}$$

where $\tilde{\theta}_3$ captures the impact of the observables directly on outcome as well as their impact on the deterministic portion of the heterogeneous coefficients (i.e., $\tilde{\theta}_3 = \theta_3 + \beta_1 + \beta_2 c_i$).[15]

---

[15]In the empirical part of this paper, I do not interact any of the observables with the indicator as I believe

Using this equation, one can consistently estimate the mean impact of receiving treatment at facility A rather than B, $\bar{\theta}_2$, since all unobservable elements have been replaced with consistent estimates of them.[16]

Within the control function, τ tells us something about the relationship between the individual-specific responsiveness to treatment at A and the decision to actually receive treatment there. A positive coefficient would indicate that persons whose observables suggest that they are unlikely to receive treatment at A, yet choose to do so, are disproportionately likely to benefit from receiving treatment there (assuming that y is a positive, desirable outcome). Thus, by examining $\hat{\tau}$ one can check the validity of the behavioral assumption underpinning the model.

3.2 Empirical Specification with Multiple Endogenous Treatment Options

This paper's primary technical innovation is to suggest a tractable means of moving from the one endogenous treatment setting described above to a polychotonous one. This requires the specification of the choice set of facilities available to each patient, as well as the process by which a facility is chosen. In addition, I must express the appropriate control function given that there will be more than one endogenous variable. As discussed below, the existing literatures on patient choice modeling and multinomial Roy models suggest straightforward ways of addressing these issues.

First, consistent with the prior literature on hospital choice modeling (Kessler and Mc-Clellan, 2000, Tay, 2003, Ho, 2006), I assume that each patient considers each facility within some radius of their home. In other words, each patient i evaluates the utility V that each of

---

it is more correct to incorporate any information about particular matching based on patient and facility characteristics into the choice function. Thus, if the aged benefited disproportionately from treatment at A, then this should already be accounted for by including age in the facility selection model.

[16]Moreover, examination of Equation (8) shows why IV estimation of Equation (2) would not be consistent. This is because even if $E[\phi^1|z] = 0$, $E[\phi^2 c|z] \neq 0$ unless strong assumptions hold about both the orthogonality of the product of the endogenous variables and their residuals and the homoskedasticity of the residuals. This is generally untrue (Heckman and Vytlacil, 1998). In contrast, the CF approach of including the residuals from the first stage and the interaction of that residual with the endogenous variable will produce consistent estimates via standard estimation techniques for dealing with f.

the different facilities j of a possible J within a specified radius would give them. Formally, I assume that this utility can be modelled as:

$$V_{ij} = m(d_{ij}, k_{ij}) + \mu_j + e_{ij}, \qquad (9)$$

where $m(d_{ij}, k_{ij})$ is a function of the distance d between the patient's zipcode and the facility's zipcode and a set of patient or facility characteristics k, μ_j is a facility fixed effect, and e_{ij} is information unobserved by the econometrician that affects the desirability of seeking treatment at j.

If the e_{ij} are independent draws from the extreme value distribution, then the utility that a patient receives from choosing a given facility is independent of its other choices, and implies that Equation (9) can be estimated via conditional logit. This assumption is common in the hospital choice literature (Capps et al., 2003, Ho, 2006), and also seems reasonable in the dialysis industry. In large part, the strong assumption of independence to the presence of irrelevant alternatives has not been deemed problematic because the combination of fairly detailed patient-level information and facility fixed effects can be expected to sop up a very large amount of heterogeneity.

Second, following estimation of the choice problem implied by Equation (9), I use the recovered coefficients to predict the likelihood that patient i chooses facility j. These predictions are then subtracted from the binary indicator variable capturing whether or not patient i actually does choose to visit facility j to produce an η_{ij} for each possible j of J.[17] Since not all facilities are within the choice set, I impose that $\eta_{ij} = 0$ for all facilities outside the specified choice radius.[18]

The multiplicity of η that the procedure above produces requires alterations to Equation (8). In particular, the nature of the interactions between the residuals and the endogenous

---

[17]This ensures that the error terms are broadly proportional in magnitude to the endogenous regressors, which may be important in small samples or non-linear settings. Moreover, it connects directly to the work done by Dahl (2002) on Roy model problems with multiple markets.

[18]This conditional logit approach departs from the approach taken in Gowrisankaran and Town (1999), who used a dichotomous discrete choice model and a non-linear function of distance to estimate whether or not a given patient chose each possible hospital.

15

variable must be specified. As shown in Luan and Sudhir (2010), without assumptions about the relationship between the error terms in the first stage models, including J endogenous variables implies that the control function should include the J residuals directly plus J^2 interaction terms. These interactions account for the possibility that the unobservable information affecting the selection of an endogenous variable disproportionately affects the responsiveness to another. In many cases, including that of Luan and Sudhir (2010), controlling for the possibility of such interrelatedness seems both reasonable and appropriate. However, in my setting, it is unduly conservative, running contrary to the assumption made in estimating the facility choice model that the error terms impacting the utilities of the different options are independent. Therefore, it is reasonable to believe that the only residual impacting the slope of a given endogenous variable is the one from its own first-stage equation. Formally, what this means is that after conditioning on the η associated with a given facility, I assume no other element in the choice problem affects the treatment effect associated with that facility.

Altogether, these assumptions imply that the control function, which took the form $\psi \eta_i + \tau \eta_i c_i$ when there was only one endogenous element, generalizes to $\sum_{j=k}^{K} \psi_j \eta_{ij} + \tau_j \eta_{ij} c_{ij}$ when there are K endogenous elements. Thus, the baseline estimating equation for patient outcomes becomes:

$$y_{ij} = f(\bar{\theta}_j c_{ij} + \overbrace{\sum_{i=k}^{K} (\psi_j \hat{\eta}_{ij} + \tau_j \hat{\eta}_{ij} c_{ij})}^{\text{control function}} + x_{ij} \tilde{\theta}_3) + \epsilon_{ij}, \tag{10}$$

where time subscripts are suppressed for the sake of concision.

3.3 Identification of Treatment Quality in the Outcome Equation

It is worth being explicit about how my CF approach relates to past treatments of multinomial selection models and their identification results. In many ways, it is highly analogous to the semi-parametric approach of Dahl (2002), which drew on intuition provided in Lee (1983). In Dahl's paper, the concern is that individuals select into states where they can expect to earn higher wages, possibly biasing coefficients on other variables. Dahl shows that the selection issue caused by this multinomial choice problem can be parsimoniously addressed using just a function of the probability that an individual would migrate to that state provided certain assumptions about the choice process are met. Formally speaking, identification requires that no element in the individual's location choice problem affects the outcome variable (in his case wage) after conditioning on the likelihood of having chosen the actual location. This overarching assumption is met by the IIA assumptions required for the conditional logit I use to estimate the facility choice model.[19]

Though relying on similar identification assumptions, it is important to note that my specification differs from Dahl (2002) in several important ways. First, whereas he uses a function of the choice probabilities themselves, I include their residuals. This difference does not meaningully change the identification approach. Second, whereas Dahl (2002) uses a bin estimator to find individuals' migration probabilties, I take advantage of a smaller set of outcomes per patient to estimate these directly using a parametric choice model. As shown in recent work (Carlson et al., 2014), the conditional logit approach and the bin approach used by Dahl (2002) are asymptotically equivalent.[20] Third, and finally, while Dahl (2002) estimates a separate selection-corrected model for each state, I include all of the endogenous variables in one equation. The location-by-location approach will be more fitting when there is considerable heterogeneity in variables' impacts across states, but the simultaneous model adopted here will be more efficient if many of the observable regressors have equivalent effects on outcomes irrespective of facility choice. That seems especially likely in this case. Thus, none of the differences in my approach significantly impacts the validity of inference.

---

[19]When such strong independence assumptions are not met, one may wish to turn to models accomodating richer correlation structure between selection and the outcome variables. These might include generalizations of the approach suggested in Dubin and McFadden (1984) and advanced in Bourguignon et al. (2007).

[20]I have cursorily explored using a bin estimator in lieu of the conditional logit model. Unfortunately, including more than zipcode and year elements in the definition of a "bin" means that few people would be within it. Thus, there would be either a high likelihood of over- or under-fitting the probability of a given individual frequenting a given facility depending on whether coarser or finer bins were used.

3.4 Inferring Determinants of Quality

Once the facility-specific average quality coefficients have been consistently estimated $(\hat{\bar{\theta}})$ using Equation (10), insight into how different market-level and facility-level factors influence treatment quality can be gained by decomposing them. This idea owes much to the structural productivity literature (Syverson, 2011), and a related approach was previously employed by Gowrisankaran and Town (1999) to analyze the impact of hospital ownership on patient mortality after controlling for unobserved condition severity.

In my decompositions, I regress estimated time invariant quality effects on the average values of market structure, the facilities' modal ownership status, and other facility-specific characteristics.[21] Thus, to understand the relationship between quality at facility j and market or facility characteristics, I estimate the following regression:

$$\hat{\bar{\theta}}_{jm} = \bar{M}_{mj}\beta + e_{jm}, \tag{11}$$

where M is a vector of market- and facility-level characteristics and m indexes markets. The impacts of the different factors are identified off of cross-sectional variation across facilities.

It is useful to think carefully about what endogeneity problems Equation (11) solves, as well as those it does not. Signally, the decomposition of the CF model estimates of facility quality is not subject to what seems like the biggest endogeneity concern: systematic co-location of facilities and the patients they are best suited to. For example, if a given local population was of unobservably good health, making them cheaper to treat, then one might expect greater than otherwise expected entry. Naive regressions of quality on market structure would then falsely suggest a stronger than "true" relationship between competition and quality. In addition, if facilities specialize, and increased competition leads to greater specialization, then the result will be raw quality estimates that are increasingly contaminated by selection effects as competition increases. The CF approach explicitly addresses both of these possible concerns as the quality estimates it produces are purged of the impact of unobserved

---

[21]I do not exploit intertemporal variation as preliminary analyses found quality to be fairly stable, and it would be difficult to precisely estimate facility-year quality effects given the sample size.

condition severity and the possibility that some facilities specialize. Thus, a regression of the estimated quality metric on the market structure proxies should be expected to consistently capture the "true" impact of competition.

One might still worry if patients were located in two wholly separate areas. In that case, the model might not fully address the relation between patients' unobservables and market structure. However, in this paper's empirical implementation, I consider an environment where the patient population is spread continuously over an area. Thus, I can exploit people's willingness to travel to identify heterogeneity in the treatment quality.

While the selection correction approach integral to my empirical model addresses my main endogeneity concern, it is possible to think of possible problems that it does not fix. In particular, consider a given facility that is of particularly high quality. One might worry that its strength would deter competitors from subsequently locating nearby. Thus, Equation (11) would return a biased representation of the competition-quality relationship. I would argue, however, that this concern is not particularly dire. In practice, such entry deterrence is unlikely to happen on a meaningful scale. Though the footprint of dialysis clinics is not enormous, especially relative to that of hospitals, the number of available locations is unlikely to be large within a given general vicinity. Therefore, the capacity to pick one's competition is limited. Moreover, given the practical importance of proximity as a driver of patient traffic, even an inferior – on average – facility could reasonably expect to steal a reasonable amount of patients within a local area. Finally, to the extent that – on the margin – competitors did try to locate away from high quality incumbents, it would tend to attenuate the impact of competition, making any finding of a positive correlation between competition and quality conservative evidence of the relationship.

4 Data Discussion & Descriptive Analysis

4.1 Data

In assessing the influence of market structure and ownership on patient outcomes, this paper relies on data obtained from the United States Renal Dialysis System (USRDS). Part of the National Institute of Diabetes and Digestive and Kidney Diseases (NIDDK), the USRDS collects and integrates data taken from a variety of surveys performed by other elements of the National Institutes of Health (NIH), Centers for Medicare and Medicaid Services (CMS), and other governmental agencies. These data are at both the patient and facility level.

The USRDS facility data previously were exploited in Wilson (2013), and include information on factors like where a given facility is located (down to the zipcode level), its ownership status (for-profit, non-profit, and a small number of cases where ownership status is unknown), and the chain with which the facility is affiliated.[22] The USRDS patient-level data provide information on age, gender, race, zipcode of residence, and how long the patient has been receiving dialysis treatment. In an effort to ensure that my results are as robust as possible, I estimate treatment models excluding those who switch treatment regimes during a given year.[23]

Within the USRDS data, several different outcome variables are available for use as proxies of facility quality. I focus on the following three: whether or not the patient died during their year of treatment; the number of days the patient was hospitalized for those episodes beginning in the year they received treatment at a given facility; and the number of days the patient spent in the intensive care unit (ICU) or cardiac care unit (CCU) beginning in the year they received treatment at a particular facility. All are factors that are akin to metrics for outcome quality used in the past health services and medical literatures on dialysis facility quality (Garg et al., 1999, Ford and Kaserman, 2000, Devereaux et al., 2002,

---

[22] As described in Wilson (2013), the facility data are somewhat noisy in regards to ownership status. The approach to cleaning the facility data is described in that paper and below in the appendix. To be considered part of a chain, the USRDS requires that there be at least 20 or more facilities with the same owner. Thus, the number of facilities associated with chains in the data is a conservative estimate of the true number.

[23] See the Appendix for details on the construction of the dataset.

Brooks et al., 2006, Zhang et al., 2011).

In addition to the USRDS data, I also exploit demographic information from the Surveillance, Epidemiology and End Results (SEER) Program, which is also affiliated with the NIH. Since ESRD grows in commonality with age, I follow Wilson (2013) and proxy for local demand for dialysis services using the county population that is over 60. Since zipcodes do not map perfectly to counties, I match each zipcode to the county it was most closely associated with (in terms of population) in the Census' ZCTA-county correspondence.

In the decomposition stage, one of the key questions of interest is the connection between facility quality and market structure. For my baseline models, I characterize market structure using the (logged) number of competitors within a certain radius. This is consistent with various past analyses of competition in retail industries (Shepard, 1993, Hosken et al., 2008). I focus on the number of facilities within 10 miles of the centrum of the zipcode a facility is located within, controlling for whether or not the facilities share the same owner as the focal facility.[24]

Table 1 shows the number of facility-year observations affiliated with each chain in the Atlanta area, while Figure 2 shows a map of the facilities' locations. The Table indicates that the overwhelming majority of facilities are affiliated with either DaVita or Fresenius. Of the chains identified in the USRDS data, only DCI operates as a non-profit. Approximately 55 percent of observations in the sample associated with independents are with for-profit facilities. The Figure suggests that the two large chains' facilities are somewhat less likely to be in the city center.

4.2 Descriptive Analysis

As noted above, in order to appropriately estimate the choice model, rules must be established for which facilities belong in each patient's choice set. An examination of the data shows that 93 percent of patients in the sample receive treatment within 20 miles of their home;

---

[24]This is broadly similar to assuming that firms' 75% service territories delineate the relevant geographic market. As discussed further below, the qualitative findings that this geographic market definition produces are robust to alternative specifications.

86 percent do so within 15 miles; and 71 percent receive care within 10 miles. Therefore, I define patients' choice sets as the larger of the set of facilities within 15 miles of their home zipcode, if they choose a facility within that radius, or all of the facilities within the radius of their chosen facility.[25]

Table 2 shows descriptive statistics at the facility level. Summary values are shown for the entire sample as well as stratified by ownership status. In addition to considering factors like the average number of patients seen and the average population over 60 in the facility's county, I also include measures for the degree of competitiveness and concentration in their area. Overall, the Table shows quite striking differences depending on ownership status. Non-profit facilities tend to be in more competitively "congested" areas. Indeed, the average number of facilities within a 10 mile radius of the centrum of a non-profit facility's zipcode is three times as high as that for a for-profit facility. However, almost none of these share a similar owner, which is consistent with the low penetration of DCI in shown in the Atlanta area. Interestingly, the average non-profit facility sees many more patients in a year than the average for-profit one, and are – on average – twice as old.

Table 3 shows descriptive statistics at the patient level for the entire sample as well as for those patients frequenting for-profit and non-profit facilities.[26] Intuitively given the evolution of the industry, a large majority of patients receive care at for-profit facilities. Somewhat less intuitively, the Table indicates quite dramatic differences in the average patient seen across ownership forms, which is in line with the findings of Zhang et al. (2011) referenced above.

The average non-profit patient is much more likely to be male, black, and a longterm sufferer of ESRD. Although not exploited in the the regressions, an analysis of the subset of data that include patients' comorbidities indicates that non-profits' patients are also more likely to self-report being a smoker and/or dependent upon alchohol. Some of these factors are typically considered risk factors. However, for-profit patients also have some characteristics typically associated with worse health outcomes. In particular, they are more likely to be

---

[25]Preliminary work with alternative rules led to similar findings.

[26]I do not provide summary values for the small number of patients frequenting facilities whose ownership status is not known in the data.

older and report suffering from diabetes.

Focusing on patient outcomes, Table 3 suggests that the average outcome for patients at non-profit facilities is superior to that for patients at for-profit facilities. Average mortality is 12 percent lower, the number of days in either the CCU or ICU is 33 percent lower, and the number of days hospitalized overall is 25 percent lower. These simple statistics would appear consistent with the conventional expectation that non-profits provide higher quality, which – as noted above – several past analyses of the dialysis sector have also found. However, the differences in the average patient described above suggest that some of the differences could in fact be at least partially attributed to for-profit facilities consistently treating sicker patients. In which case, for-profits' average performance may only look worse before controlling for patient severity.

All of this suggests that it is quite important to control for the possibility of systemmatic selection of treating facility before making any conclusions. Therefore, I now turn to more formal methods of inferring the impact of different facility and market characteristics on treatment quality.

5 Does Patient Selection Matter?

For each of the three outcome variables – mortality, the (logged) days of "serious" hospitalization, and the (logged) overall number of days hospitalized, I estimate OLS, facility FE, IV, and CF models. In other words, I estimate linear versions of Equation (2) for these outcomes, dealing with the possibility of heterogeneous coefficients in different ways.

As discussed above, the IV and CF models both rely on a first stage conditional logit model of the likelihood that a given patient chooses a given facility.[27] The choice models include facility fixed effects as well as a quadratic function of distance, the interaction of

---

[27]To be clear, for the IV model, I simply replace the endogenous variables with the predicted likelihood of choosing each facility. In practice, the predicted probabilities were even more collinear, after including the many additional covariates, than the binary indicator variables, which prevented me from estimating the "qualities" of certain facilities in the IV models. For this reason, I have fewer facility-quality IV "observations" to be decomposed.

distance with patient age, the interaction of years of hemodialysis treatment with distance, and the interaction between the disease causing the patient's ESRD and the size of the facility (in terms of dialysis stations). All of the distance terms – which are the excluded variables in the outcome models – are precisely identified and of reasonable sign. The coefficient estimates for the choice model can be found in Table B-1 in the Appendix. Overall, the model does a good job of predicting in sample behavior insofar as the center with the highest predicted likelihood of being selected is actually chosen almost 40% of the time. This seems quite high given that the average patient has over 10 choices to pick from.

Tables 4, 5, and 6 show the effects of the patient-level variables on mortality, the number of days in the ICU or CCU, and total number of days hospitalized, respectively. To address the likelihood of irregular standard errors, I bootstrap with 500 replications, stratifying by facility. The resulting estimates for the impact of most of the various patient-level factors are all of reasonable signs and economic magnitude. Moreover, they are broadly consistent with the prior literature. For example, I find that older, male, and white individuals tend to have more negative health outcomes.

More interestingly, although of relatively small absolute magnitude, the differences in estimated coefficients across models are of non-trivial economic importance. For example, the 0.03 difference in the IV and CF coefficients on white in the mortality models is equivalent to 20 percent of the unconditional likelihood of death. The variation in patient characteristic coefficients across models supports the hypothesis that different facilities may target, or be viewed especially favorably by, different groups. Possibly relatedly, I consistently find that the statistical precision of the estimated impacts of disease-related factors is much lower for the IV and CF models. This may indicate that these factors play heavily into patients' selection of different facilities, and that once modeled in the choice of treating location, are no longer as consistently meaningful to outcomes in their own right. Per the logic behind Hausman tests, such differences in the signs and statistical significances of the different estimates would suggest that greater emphasis be placed on the more generally unbiased CF results.[28]

[28]I explored whether formal Hausman tests could be used to draw inferences about the appropriateness of the different metrics. Unfortunately, though not surprisingly, the test results were not well-defined, and thus

The potential importance of non-random selection, and therefore the probable superiority of the CF estimates, can also be seen by focusing on differences in the estimated quality effects themselves. However, it must be noted that the IV and – especially – CF quality estimates contain a number of dramatic outliers across outcome variables. Therefore, I winsorize those data series beyond the 10th percentile on both ends of the distribution. Descriptive statistics for the different quality estimates can be seen in Table 7. The very high degree of variability in the CF models may indicate the importance of the separately estimated individual-facility match effects, which could lead to more extreme estimated values of the average effect in small samples. It is important, however, to note that while perhaps noisy, the recovered average effect coefficients are unbiased estimates of the true parameters.

First, some sense of the magnitude of the differences across methods, as well as their lack of correlation, can be seen in Figure 3, which shows scatter plots of the facility quality estimates for the number days in the ICU/CCU quality for the CF model compared to the to the IV and FE models. As noted, the figures indicate that the methods that account for selection produce substantially more dispersed estimates than the FE model. More interestingly, the importance of controlling for selection can be seen in the fact that facilities' estimated quality effects are surprisingly uncorrelated as seen in both the Figures and Table 8, which shows the correlation matrix for all of the different facility quality estimates. However, within estimation method, facilities' estimated qualities tend to be fairly correlated.[29]

Second, not only do different estimation approaches produce observably different estimates, but traditional specification choice metrics consistently indicate that the CF models are preferable to more parsimonious alternatives. For example, following Petrin and Train (2010), I perform Wald tests of the joint insignificance of the control function elements and find that the null is rejected at the 1% level for all models. Thus, they do seem to be capturing important elements about patients' outcomes.

The final and most direct test of the CF model is to consider whether the coefficient estimates on the terms in the control function make intuitive sense. As discussed above, the

---

cannot be used to infer anything about the appropriateness of the different models (Small and Hsiao, 1985).

[29]The Table uses the same winsorized IV estimates as in the correlation table.

interaction terms capture the relationship between the heterogeneous impact of receiving treatment at a given location and the choice to receive treatment there. Since outcomes are negative in these models, one would expect to find negative coefficients on the interaction terms. This would show that if patients' were highly unlikely to choose a given treating facility, yet ended up receiving treatment there, the choice would be associated with lower expected mortality, fewer days in the ICU/CCU, and/or less days hospitalized. Although the individual estimated coefficients are heterogeous, summary statistics of the estimates show that they are negative on average; this is true for both the raw estimates and the winsorized values.[30] The included residual terms also provide some intuitive results. Their coefficients are – on average – negative, which indicates that choosing to go to a non-predicted facility is associated with better outcomes.

Overall, the evidence from the different treatment models lends support to the idea of selection based not just on condition severity but also heterogeneous response to treatments. However, the question of the practical importance of accounting for such endogeneity when considering the relationship between market structure and quality remains.

6   What Determines Facility Quality?

To explore the practical implications of facility selection on the relationship between market structure and mean quality, I present two different tables of results.[31] Table 9 shows decompositions of the CF model quality estimates on simple proxies for market structure and organizational characteristics, while Table 10 shows similar decompositions using the quality estimates from FE and IV models. I again adjust for the likelihood of non-standard error structures by bootstrapping (500 replications), and continue to use the winsorized data series described above.

Because of the small number of observations, I include a very parsimonious set of regres-

---

[30]Moreover, weighting by relative statistical precision (in this case, the inverse of the coefficient of variation) does not alter this conclusion. This is always true for the winsorized values, though one raw series has a positive mean when weights are employed.

[31]Table B-2 shows descriptive statistics for the included variables in the Appendix.

sors in the decompositions. My baseline approach to accounting for market structure is to use the logged sum of all facilities in the area (i.e., including the facility of interest), and the share of facilities in the area affiliated with the facility's owner. In other words, if a given facility j faces four other nearby dialysis providers, and two of these are affiliated with j's owner, then the share variable's value would be 60%.[32] I also include a binary indicator for whether or not the facility has non-profit status, and a limited set of chain identifiers that account for the possibility that Davita and/or Fresenius behave differently than the mass of all other facilities.[33]

Table 9 tells a consistent story about the relationship between average treatment quality and concentration. As the number of nearby facilities under the same ownership increases, the facility's mean quality declines by a statistically and economically significant amount for all three outcome metrics. Moreover, given the estimated coefficient values, the results also imply that an increase in the number of non-affiliated facilities – i.e., increased competition – improves quality for a facility in most markets in the data. This is because although the coefficient on the logged sum of facilities is positive, each additional non-affiliated facility reduces the share of local facilities under the control of the same owner as the facility of interest.

The non-linear relationship between market structure and quality can be seen in Figure 4. Each panel in the Figure shows the estimated impact on quality of different market structures. The X axes indicate the total number of facilities, while the Y axes account for the number of these facilities associated with the owner of the facility in question. Thus, Panel B shows that for approximately the average facility, which faces 14 competitors of which four are affiliated, an acquisition of a fifth additional facility would lead to a 28% percent increase in the expected number of days spent in the ICU/CCU, holding constant the total number of nearby facilities.

In addition to suggesting a positive relationship between quality and competition, which

---

[32] As described in further detail below, the qualitative results from this specification are robust to other parameterizations of market structure.

[33] I do not specify which chain effect estimate is for which chain.

is strongly consistent with economic theory (Gaynor, 2006), the results demonstrate the importance of accounting for patient selection for several factors. Table 10 shows how different types of selection impact different types of treatment effects. The FE models use estimates of the average effect of treatment on the treated without adjusting for unobserved condition severity. Insofar as they indicate little to no relationship between competition and quality, their results are in line with the hypothesis that the selection of sicker patients to higher quality facilities will lead to downwardly biased estimates of quality. Thus, if competition is correlated with higher quality, the estimated impact of competition will be biased down.

The IV models also use quality estimates that reflect the impact of treatment on the treated, but do so after conditioning out unobserved patient severity. Thus, they indicate how changes in market structure impact average quality when patients optimize on their heterogenous match with different facilities. Their results show broadly similar qualitative patterns to those from the CF models, but with markedly smaller magnitudes. For example, whereas the CF models predicted that acquiring one additional facility would increase the number of days in the ICU/CCU by 28% for the average facility, the IV model would predict only a 3% increase. Such attenuation in the estimates indicates that different facilities' have different specializations, even within a given company's network, which lead to smaller quality effects than than the change in the average treatment effects presented in the CF model would suggest.

Although in line with most papers on hospital competition (Gaynor and Town, 2011), my finding that competition fosters better average quality is not consistent with either of the most recent economic papers on the dialysis industry. Grieco and McDevitt (2012) find a non-monotonic relationship between competition and average quality, with monopolists providing the highest quality of care, while Cutler et al. (2012) find no connection between concentration and patient care. I believe that our disparate findings can be reconciled in a variety of ways.

First, Grieco and McDevitt (2012) make the implicit assumption – perhaps as a result of data limitations – that all facilities compete on equal grounds irrespective of ownership.

In contrast, I accomodate the existence and substantial importance of chains, allowing for facilities affiliated with the same chain to have different impacts than those affiliated with other owners. When I estimate models that treat all facilities equally, I am able to produce results more qualitatively similar to theirs insofar as I find that average quality deteriorates in the presence of additional outlets. This can be seen in Table B-3 in the Appendix.

Second, the metrics that Grieco and McDevitt (2012) and Cutler et al. (2012) use for quality are "raw" and, thus, broadly comparable to my FE estimates. Therefore, if the methods that the different papers employ to address the endogeneity of quality and market structure do not fully account account for the importance of patient selection, then their estimates of the impact of market structure may not be unbiased.

In addition to my results' implications for the relationship between average quality and competition, the decomposition of the CF estimates of quality suggest that the average quality of non-profit facilities may be inferior to that of for-profit facilities. However, this inference should be approached with caution given the very small number of non-profit facilities within the data and the imprecision of the point estimates. Nevertheless, this raises interesting questions about evaluating the role of profit status in care provision insofar as most prior work implies that for-profit facilities are more efficient (Held and Pauly, 1983, Wilson, 2013). I am hopeful that future work may shed new light on this issue.

Overall, the results of my decomposition of the CF facility quality estimates strongly support the mainstream opinion of economists that competition is positively associated with treatment quality. Moreover, I found this result robust to alternative specifications. Evidence of this can be seen in Tables B-4 and B-5 in the Appendix, which show the results of similar models where facility-level observations are weighted by the number of patients seen at that facility, when the market-structure measures are based on 8-mile radius instead of a 10-mile one, and when the market structure variables are replaced with level measures normalized by the county population over 60.[34] Across all of these different models, I find highly similar

---

[34] As suggested in Solon et al. (2013), I considered whether weighting plausibly addresses the possibility of heteroskedastic errors across the different facilities. The results of the modified Breusch-Pagan test they describe do suggest that one would typically reject the assumption of homoskedastic errors across facilities. However, the magnitudes are quite similar across models.

qualitative results.[35]

7 Conclusion

In this paper, I focus on how selection concerns complicate health outcome modeling. To address this problem, I develop a control function estimator that addresses not only the standard concern about unobservable variation in condition severity but also heterogeneous responsiveness to treatment. The modeling framework is then applied to dialysis patient data from the USRDS.

Specification tests suggest that not only is "traditional" selection a significant problem in identifying the average quality of different facilities, but so too is heterogeneous responsiveness to treatment. Decomposing the estimates of treatment facility quality obtained from the control function model, I find evidence consistent with the hypothesis that competition fosters higher quality care. I also find some evidence that for-profit facilities' average quality of care is no worse, and perhaps better, than that of non-profits. Taken together, the results indicate that there can be anticompetitive implications from increased concentration even when prices are administratively determined. This buttresses the ongoing concern of antitrust authorities about the sharp increase in concentration in the dialysis industry as well as health care markets more broadly (Dafny, 2013).

Going forward, the paper's finding that idiosyncratic matching is economically and statistically important even in an ostensibly undifferentiated service market like dialysis suggests that it is a phenomenon that should be considered in other settings. This is especially the case given that accounting for it in the dialysis industry appears to explain the mixed results in the prior literature. As richer data on outcomes as well as choices become available, it will be interesting to explore whether similarly significant levels of idiosyncratic fit are found for other industries or markets.

---

[35]In addition, I experimented with including average county population to address concerns that the market structure variables were simply capturing something about density. The variable had no meaningful impact. Finally, I experimented with using the logged sum of affiliated and unaffiliated centers nearby as proxies for market structure. This approach produced qualitatively similar results.

References

Beaudry, Paul, David A Green, and Benjamin Sand, "Spill-overs from good jobs," Technical Report, National Bureau of Economic Research 2007.

_ , Mark Doms, and Ethan Lewis, "Should the personal computer be considered a technological revolution? evidence from US metropolitan areas," *Journal of Political Economy*, 2010, *118* (5), 988–1036.

Berry, Steven, James Levinsohn, and Ariel Pakes, "Automobile prices in market equilibrium," *Econometrica: Journal of the Econometric Society*, 1995, pp. 841–890.

Bourguignon, François, Martin Fournier, and Marc Gurgand, "Selection bias corrections based on the multinomial logit model: Monte Carlo comparisons," *Journal of Economic Surveys*, 2007, *21* (1), 174–205.

Brooks, J.M., C.P. Irwin, L.G. Hunsicker, M.J. Flanigan, E.A. Chrischilles, and J.F. Pendergast, "Effect of Dialysis Center Profit-Status on Patient Survival: A Comparison of Risk-Adjustment and Instrumental Variable Approaches," *Health Services Research*, 2006, *41* (6), 2267–2289.

Capps, Cory, David Dranove, and Mark Satterthwaite, "Competition and market power in option demand markets," *RAND Journal of Economics*, 2003, pp. 737–763.

Card, David, "Estimating the Return to Schooling: Progress on Some Persistent Econometric Problems," *Econometrica*, 2001, *69* (5), 1127–1160.

Carlson, J., L. Dafny, B. Freeborn, P. Ippolito, and B. Wendling, "Economics at the FTC: Physician Acquisitions, Standard Essential Patents, and Accuracy of Credit Reporting," *Review of Industrial Organization*, 2014.

Cutler, David, Leemore Dafny, and Christopher Ody, "Competition in Quality: The Case of U.S. Dialysis Clinics," *mimeo*, 2012.

Dafny, Leemore, "Hospital Industry Consolidation - Still more to come?," *New England Journal of Medicine*, 2013.

Dahl, Gordon B, "Mobility and the return to education: Testing a Roy model with multiple markets," *Econometrica*, 2002, *70* (6), 2367–2420.

Devereaux, PJ, H.J. Schünemann, N. Ravindran, M. Bhandari, A.X. Garg, P.T.L. Choi, B.J.B. Grant, T. Haines, C. Lacchetti, B. Weaver et al., "Comparison of mortality between private for-profit and private not-for-profit hemodialysis centers," *JAMA: the journal of the American Medical Association*, 2002, *288* (19), 2449–2457.

Dubin, Jeffrey A and Daniel L McFadden, "An econometric analysis of residential electric appliance holdings and consumption," *Econometrica: Journal of the Econometric Society*, 1984, pp. 345–362.

Dustmann, Christian and Costas Meghir, "Wages, experience and seniority," *The Review of Economic Studies*, 2005, *72* (1), 77–108.

Farley, D.O., "Effects of Competition of Dialysis Facility Service Levels and Patient Selection," RAND Corporation Ph.D. Dissertation 1993.

Fields, R., "'God help you. You're on Dialysis.'," *The Atlantic*, December 2010.

_ , "In Dialysis, Life-Saving Care at Great Risk and Cost," *ProPublica*, November 2010.

Ford, J.M. and D.L. Kaserman, "Ownership structure and the quality of medical care: evidence from the dialysis industry," *Journal of Economic Behavior & Organization*, 2000, *43* (3), 279–293.

Garg, P.P., K.D. Frick, M. Diener-West, and N.R. Powe, "Effect of the ownership of dialysis facilities on patients' survival and referral for transplantation," *New England Journal of Medicine*, 1999, *341* (22), 1653–1660.

Gaynor, M. and R.J. Town, "Competition in health care markets," Technical Report, National Bureau of Economic Research 2011.

_ , **H. Seider, and W.B. Vogt**, "The volume-outcome effect, scale economies, and learning-by-doing," *American Economic Review*, 2005, pp. 243–247.

Gaynor, Martin, "What do we know about competition and quality in health care markets?," Technical Report, National Bureau of Economic Research 2006.

Geweke, J., G. Gowrisankaran, and R.J. Town, "Bayesian Inference for Hospital Quality in a Selection Model," *Econometrica*, 2003, *71* (4), 1215–1238.

Gowrisankaran, G. and R.J. Town, "Estimating the quality of care in hospitals using instrumental variables," *Journal of Health Economics*, 1999, *18* (6), 747–767.

Grieco, P.L.E. and R.C. McDevitt, "Productivity and Quality in Health Care: Evidence from the Dialysis Industry," *mimeo*, 2012.

Heckman, J., "Dummy exogenous variables in a simulation equation system," *Econometrica*, 1978, *46*.

Heckman, James and Edward Vytlacil, "Instrumental variables methods for the correlated random coefficient model: Estimating the average rate of return to schooling when the return is correlated with schooling," *Journal of Human Resources*, 1998, pp. 974–987.

Held, P.J. and M.V. Pauly, "Competition and efficiency in the end stage renal disease program," *Journal of Health Economics*, 1983, *2* (2), 95–118.

Henderson, LW, "Heterogeneity of the cardiovascular response to hemofiltration.," *Kidney international*, 1986, *29* (4), 901–907.

Ho, Katherine, "The welfare effects of restricted hospital choice in the US medical care market," *Journal of Applied Econometrics*, 2006, *21* (7), 1039–1079.

Hosken, D.S., R.S. McMillan, and C.T. Taylor, "Retail gasoline pricing: What do we know?," *International Journal of Industrial Organization*, 2008, *26* (6), 1425–1436.

Jones, Katherine R, "Variations in the hemodialysis treatment process," *Clinical Nursing Research*, 1992, *1* (1), 50–66.

Kagari, A, Y Bar-Khaym, Z Schafer, and M Fainaru, "Heterogeneity in Peritoneal Transport during Continuous Ambulatory Peritoneal Dialysis and Its Impact on Ultraf iltration, Loss of Macromolecules and Plasma Level of Proteins, Lipids and Lipoproteins," *Nephron*, 1993, *63* (1), 32–42.

Katz, Michael L, "Provider competition and healthcare quality: More bang for the buck?," *International Journal of Industrial Organization*, 2013.

Kessler, D.P. and M.B. McClellan, "Is Hospital Competition Socially Wasteful?," *Quarterly Journal of Economics*, 2000, pp. 577–615.

Lee, D.K.K., G.M. Chertow, and S.A. Zenios, "Reexploring Differences among For-Profit and Nonprofit Dialysis Providers," *Health Services Research*, 2010, *45* (3), 633–646.

Lee, L.F., "Unionism and wage rates: A simultaneous equations model with qualitative and limited dependent variables," *International economic review*, 1978, *19* (2), 415–433.

Lee, Lung-Fei, "Generalized econometric models with selectivity," *Econometrica: Journal of the Econometric Society*, 1983, pp. 507–512.

Liu, Xuepeng, Mary E Lovely, and Jan Ondrich, "The location decisions of foreign investors in China: Untangling the effect of wages using a control function approach," *The Review of Economics and Statistics*, 2010, *92* (1), 160–166.

Luan, Y.J. and K. Sudhir, "Forecasting marketing-mix responsiveness for new products," *Journal of Marketing Research*, 2010, *47* (3), 444–457.

Petrin, A. and K. Train, "A control function approach to endogeneity in consumer choice models," *Journal of Marketing Research*, 2010, *47* (1), 3–13.

Phrommintikul, Arintaya, Steven Joseph Haas, Maros Elsik, and Henry Krum, "Mortality and target haemoglobin concentrations in anaemic patients with chronic kidney disease treated with erythropoietin: a meta-analysis," *The Lancet*, 2007, *369* (9559), 381 – 388.

Pozniak, A.S., R.A. Hirth, J. Banaszak-Holl, and J.R.C. Wheeler, "Predictors of Chain Acquisition among Independent Dialysis Facilities," *Health Services Research*, 2010, *45* (2), 476–496.

Ramanarayanan, S. and J. Snyder, "Reputation and Firm Performance: Evidence from the Dialysis Industry," *mimeo*, 2012.

Relman, A.S. and D. Rennie, "Treatment of End-Stage Renal Disease," *New England Journal of Medicine*, 1980, *303* (17), 996–998.

Romano, P.S. and R. Mutter, "The evolving science of quality measurement for hospitals: Implications for studies of competition and consolidation," *International Journal of Health Care Finance and Economics*, 2004, *4* (2), 131–157.

Salop, Steven C, "Monopolistic competition with outside goods," *The Bell Journal of Economics*, 1979, pp. 141–156.

Schaefer, J-H, F Jochimsen, F Keller, K Wegscheider, and A Distler, "Outcome prediction of acute renal failure in medical intensive care," *Intensive care medicine*, 1991, *17* (1), 19–24.

Schiffl, Helmut, Susanne M. Lang, and Rainald Fischer, "Daily Hemodialysis and the Outcome of Acute Renal Failure," *New England Journal of Medicine*, 2002, *346* (5), 305–310. PMID: 11821506.

Shaked, Avner and John Sutton, "Relaxing price competition through product differentiation," *The Review of Economic Studies*, 1982, pp. 3–13.

Shepard, A., "Contractual form, retail price, and asset characteristics in gasoline retailing," *RAND Journal of Economics*, 1993, *24* (1), 58–77.

Small, Kenneth A and Cheng Hsiao, "Multinomial logit specification tests," *International Economic Review*, 1985, *26* (3), 619–627.

Solon, Gary, Steven J Haider, and Jeffrey Wooldridge, "What Are We Weighting For?," Technical Report, National Bureau of Economic Research 2013.

Syverson, C., "What Determines Productivity?," *Journal of Economic Literature*, 2011, *49* (2), 326–365.

Tay, A., "Assessing competition in hospital care markets: the importance of accounting for quality differentiation," *RAND Journal of Economics*, 2003, pp. 786–814.

Terza, J.V., A. Basu, and P.J. Rathouz, "Two-stage residual inclusion estimation: addressing endogeneity in health econometric modeling," *Journal of Health Economics*, 2008, *27* (3), 531–543.

— , **W.D. Bradford, and C.E. Dismuke**, "The use of linear instrumental variables methods in health services research and health economics: a cautionary note," *Health Services Research*, 2008, *43* (3), 1102–1120.

Train, K., *Discrete choice methods with simulation*, Cambridge Univ Pr, 2003.

USRDS, "United States Renal Data System Annual Report," Technical Report, United States Renal Data System 2011.

Varkevisser, M., S.A. van der Geest, and F.T. Schut, "Do patients choose hospitals with high quality ratings? Empirical evidence from the market for angioplasty in the Netherlands," *Journal of Health Economics*, 2012, *31* (2), 371–378.

Wilson, N.E., "For-Profit Status & Industry Evolution in Health Care Markets: Evidence from the Dialysis Industry," *Federal Trade Commission, mimeo*, 2013.

Zhang, Y., D.J. Cotter, and M. Thamer, "The effect of dialysis chains on mortality among patients receiving hemodialysis," *Health Services Research*, 2011, *46* (3), 747–767.

Figures

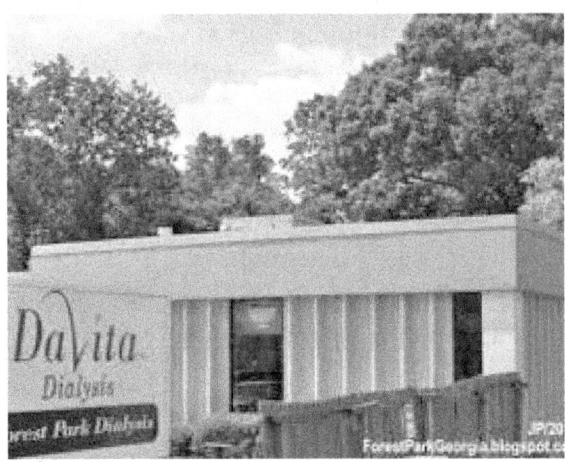

Figure 1: Example of a Dialysis Facility

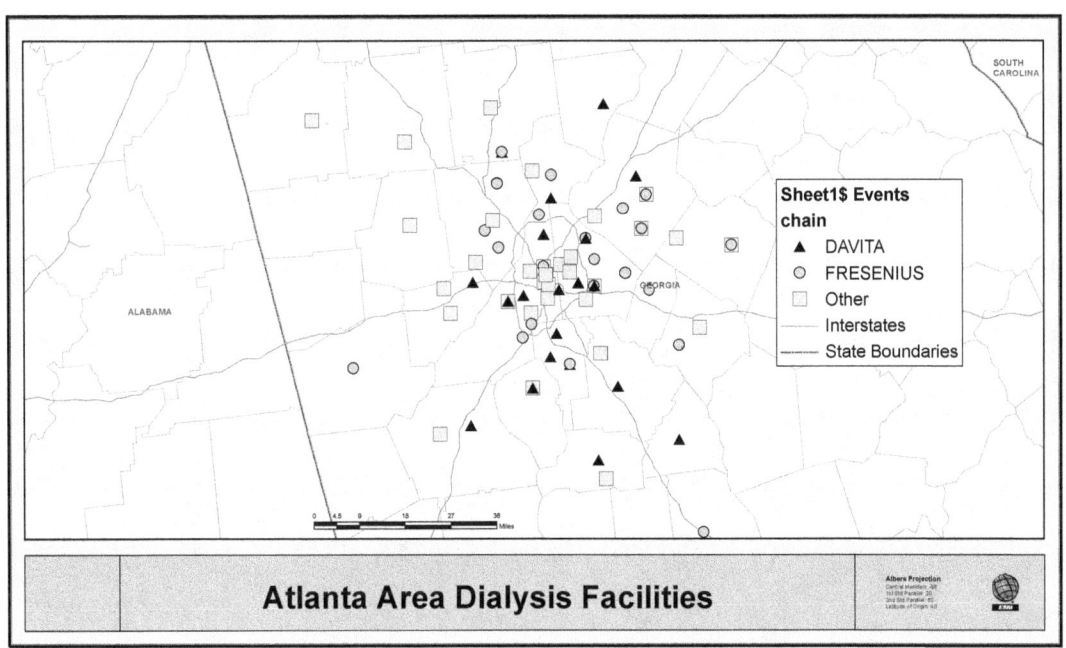

Figure 2: Chain Locations

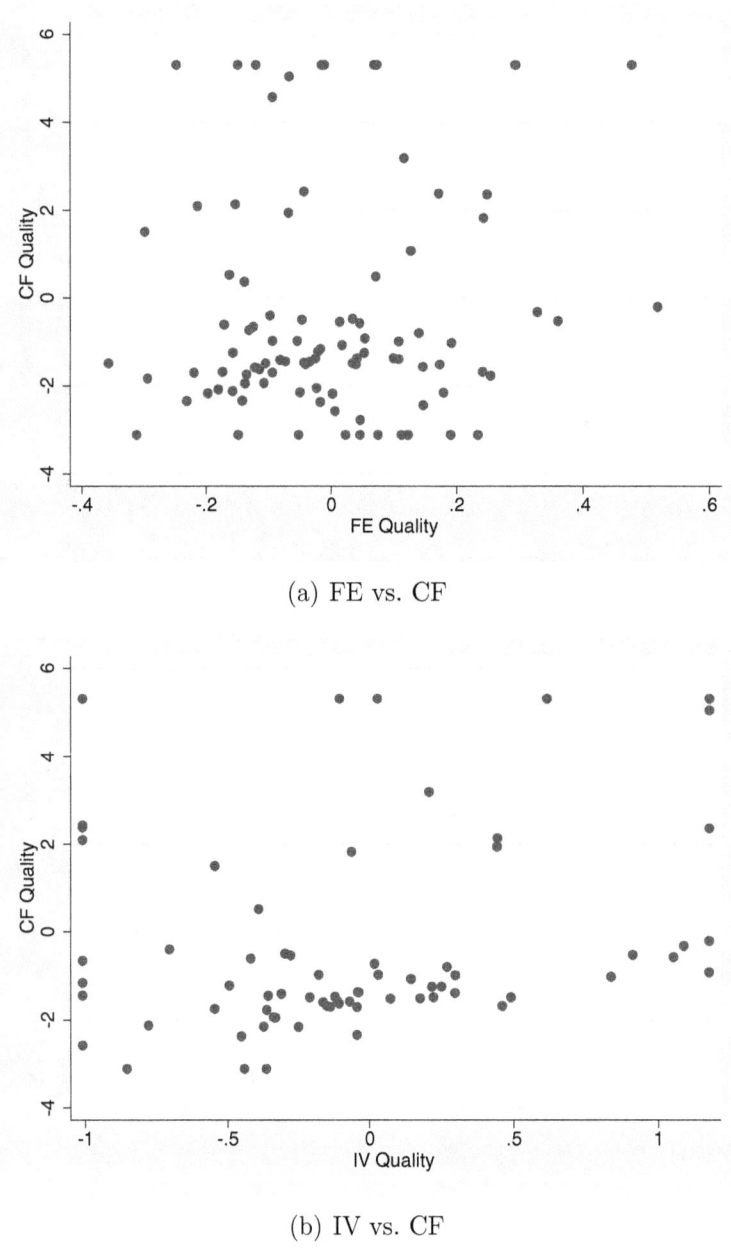

(a) FE vs. CF

(b) IV vs. CF

Figure 3: Comparison of Facility Effects on Days in CCU/ICU.

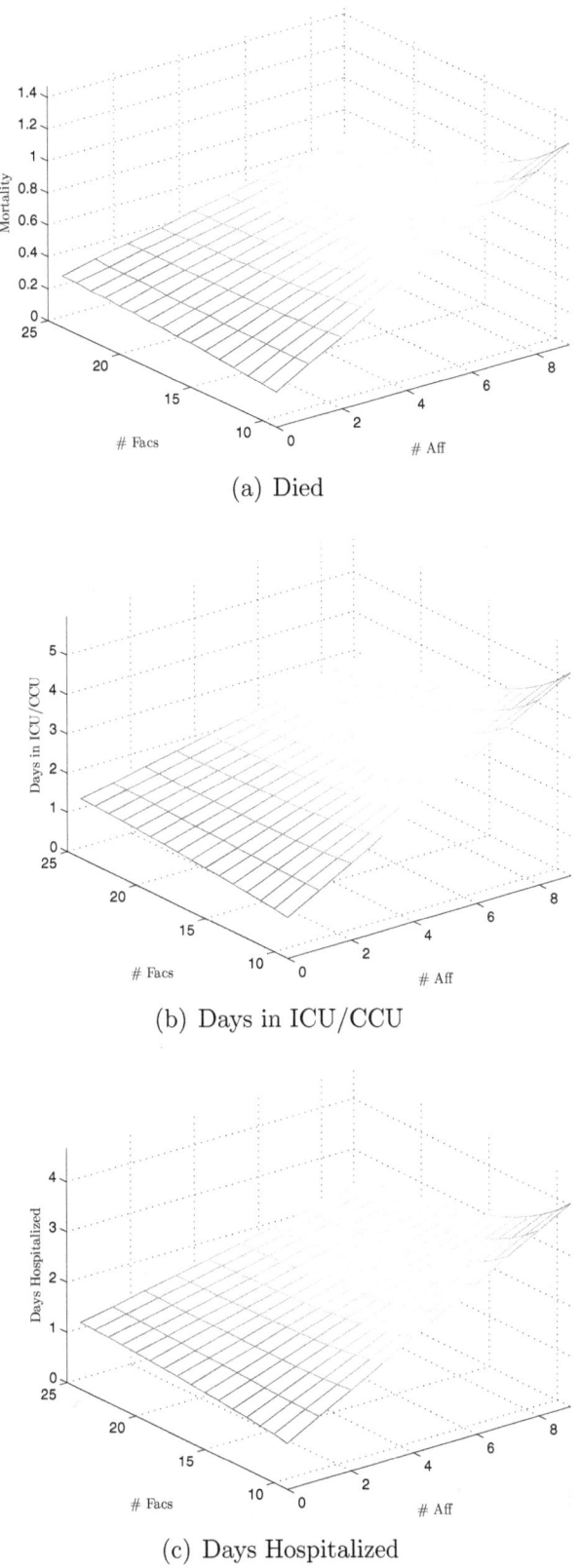

(a) Died

(b) Days in ICU/CCU

(c) Days Hospitalized

Figure 4: Impact of Market Structure on Quality.

Tables

Table 1: Brands and Ownership Structure of Facilities

Chain	Obs	Percent
Davita	7,091	29.35
DCI	1,065	4.41
Fresenius	6,004	24.85
Gambro	1,548	6.41
NRA	164	0.68
NRI	410	1.7
RCG	249	1.03
Independent	7,629	31.58
Total	24,160	100

Table 2: Variation in Facility Characteristics Across Ownership Types

	Total			For-profit			Non-profit			
	Obs	Mean	SD	Obs	Mean	SD	Obs	Mean	SD	T-Stat
Nearby Facilities	451	14.91	12.78	410	13.46	12.16	35	28.97	9.85	-8.76
Same Owner	451	3.38	4.89	410	3.58	5.07	35	1.71	1.51	5.21
Different Owner	451	11.53	10.46	410	9.88	9.11	35	27.26	9.27	-10.66
Facility Age	451	11.26	8.30	410	10.22	7.60	35	22.29	8.48	-8.14
Population > 60	451	66275	42211	410	63760	42368	35	91622	33685	-4.59
Patients	451	260.80	312.33	410	232.04	133.99	35	573.29	978.69	-2.06

Table 3: Variation in Patient Characteristics Across Ownership Types

	Obs	Total Mean	SD	Obs	For-profit Mean	SD	Obs	Non-profit Mean	SD	T-Stat
Male	24160	0.54	0.50	19672	0.52	0.50	4013	0.57	0.50	-4.90
Black	24160	0.68	0.47	19672	0.63	0.48	4013	0.89	0.32	-42.53
White	24160	0.28	0.45	19672	0.33	0.47	4013	0.07	0.25	49.78
Age	24160	5.78	1.42	19672	5.86	1.42	4013	5.34	1.37	21.85
Length of Treatment	24160	0.35	0.41	19672	0.34	0.39	4013	0.45	0.47	-14.61
Died	24160	0.14	0.35	19672	0.14	0.35	4013	0.13	0.34	1.74
Days in ICU/CCU	24160	2.79	7.88	19672	2.97	8.18	4013	2.02	6.40	8.15
Days in hospital	24160	9.75	20.48	19672	10.37	21.34	4013	7.28	16.16	10.39
1(Diabetic)	12941	0.44	0.50	10671	0.46	0.50	1997	0.39	0.49	6.19
1(Smoker)	12941	0.06	0.23	10671	0.04	0.20	1997	0.15	0.36	-13.03
1(Alcoholism)	12941	0.02	0.15	10671	0.01	0.10	1997	0.10	0.30	-13.48

Table 4: Model of Treatment Outcomes: Mortality

	OLS b/se	FE b/se	IV b/se	CF b/se
Age	-0.071***	-0.068***	-0.071***	-0.071***
	0.01	0.01	0.01	0.01
Age2	0.009***	0.009***	0.009***	0.009***
	0.001	0.001	0.001	0.001
Years Treated	-0.094***	-0.093***	-0.095***	-0.094***
	0.024	0.025	0.025	0.025
Age*Years Treated	0.027***	0.027***	0.027***	0.028***
	0.005	0.005	0.005	0.005
Male	0.007	0.006	0.007	0.006
	0.004	0.004	0.004	0.004
Black	-0.002	-0.003	-0.006	-0.006
	0.011	0.011	0.011	0.012
White	0.038**	0.042***	0.037**	0.040**
	0.012	0.012	0.012	0.012
Diabetes DG	0.231***	0.236***	0.42	0.017
	0.031	0.053	0.484	1.396
Hypertension DG	0.195***	0.199***	0.384	-0.021
	0.03	0.053	0.484	1.396
Gloeruloneph DG	0.175***	0.183***	0.365	-0.036
	0.029	0.052	0.483	1.395
Cystic Kidney DG	0.153***	0.160**	0.342	-0.06
	0.033	0.054	0.484	1.396
Other Urologic DG	0.169***	0.178**	0.361	-0.041
	0.035	0.057	0.483	1.395
Other Cause DG	0.262***	0.269***	0.453	0.05
	0.03	0.053	0.484	1.396
Unknown Cause DG	0.217***	0.223***	0.41	0.006
	0.032	0.054	0.485	1.395
Missing DG	0.265*	0.274*	0.46	0.085
	0.114	0.118	0.495	1.399
Facility Effects	No	Yes	Yes	Yes
Patient Residence FE	Yes	Yes	Yes	Yes
Year FE	Yes	Yes	Yes	Yes
N	24160	24160	24160	24160
r2	0.184	0.188	0.187	0.194

* $p<0.10$, ** $p<0.05$, *** $p<0.01$. All standard errors were bootstrapped, stratifying by facility. The model was estimated without a constant, and there was no excluded disease category. The excluded racial category is all races other than white or black. Patient residence FE are fixed effects for all patient zipcodes associated with at least 150 patients. To account for any remaining variation, I also include a complete set of patient county fixed effects.

Table 5: Model of Treatment Outcomes: (Logged) Days in ICU/CCU

	OLS b/se	FE b/se	IV b/se	CF b/se
Age	-0.045	-0.023	-0.048	-0.036
	0.03	0.031	0.031	0.031
Age2	0.015***	0.013***	0.015***	0.014***
	0.003	0.003	0.003	0.003
Years Treated	0.562***	0.551***	0.565***	0.545***
	0.063	0.062	0.063	0.062
Age*Years Treated	-0.092***	-0.087***	-0.093***	-0.086***
	0.012	0.011	0.012	0.011
Male	-0.030*	-0.023	-0.028*	-0.024
	0.013	0.013	0.013	0.014
Black	0.130***	0.139***	0.129***	0.150***
	0.027	0.027	0.028	0.029
White	0.200***	0.220***	0.195***	0.222***
	0.029	0.03	0.03	0.032
Diabetes DG	-0.341***	-0.042	0.081	4.473
	0.086	0.175	1.235	4.387
Hypertension DG	-0.411***	-0.122	0.01	4.393
	0.084	0.174	1.235	4.388
Gloeruloneph DG	-0.438***	-0.12	-0.009	4.394
	0.082	0.175	1.237	4.388
Cystic Kidney DG	-0.601***	-0.307	-0.176	4.22
	0.094	0.182	1.236	4.388
Other Urologic DG	-0.507***	-0.203	-0.077	4.322
	0.098	0.186	1.237	4.389
Other Cause DG	-0.348***	-0.046	0.077	4.465
	0.084	0.175	1.235	4.388
Unknown Cause DG	-0.393***	-0.081	0.041	4.434
	0.087	0.175	1.236	4.388
Missing DG	-0.491	-0.226	-0.053	4.357
	0.32	0.358	1.288	4.419
Facility Effects	No	Yes	Yes	Yes
Patient Residence FE	Yes	Yes	Yes	Yes
Year FE	Yes	Yes	Yes	Yes
N	24160	24160	24160	24160
r2	0.284	0.297	0.289	0.305

* $p<0.10$, ** $p<0.05$, *** $p<0.01$. All standard errors were bootstrapped, stratifying by facility. The model was estimated without a constant, and there was no excluded disease category. The excluded racial category is all races other than white or black. Patient residence FE are fixed effects for all patient zipcodes associated with at least 150 patients. To account for any remaining variation, I also include a complete set of patient county fixed effects.

Table 6: Model of Treatment Outcomes: (Logged) Days Hospitalized

	OLS b/se	FE b/se	IV b/se	CF b/se
Age	-0.180***	-0.149***	-0.183***	-0.168***
	0.044	0.044	0.044	0.045
Age2	0.034***	0.031***	0.035***	0.033***
	0.004	0.004	0.004	0.004
Years Treated	1.246***	1.200***	1.252***	1.192***
	0.093	0.093	0.093	0.094
Age*Years Treated	-0.185***	-0.174***	-0.186***	-0.172***
	0.017	0.017	0.017	0.017
Male	-0.104***	-0.079***	-0.104***	-0.080***
	0.019	0.02	0.02	0.02
Black	0.398***	0.394***	0.390***	0.405***
	0.041	0.042	0.043	0.045
White	0.527***	0.549***	0.522***	0.549***
	0.043	0.044	0.045	0.047
Diabetes DG	-0.520***	-0.127	1.347	3.513
	0.126	0.26	1.683	5.399
Hypertension DG	-0.729***	-0.352	1.132	3.286
	0.123	0.26	1.683	5.399
Gloeruloneph DG	-0.721***	-0.3	1.152	3.339
	0.122	0.26	1.684	5.397
Cystic Kidney DG	-0.890***	-0.492	0.983	3.157
	0.139	0.27	1.684	5.4
Other Urologic DG	-0.912***	-0.498	0.969	3.163
	0.142	0.271	1.685	5.399
Other Cause DG	-0.560***	-0.156	1.307	3.477
	0.123	0.262	1.683	5.397
Unknown Cause DG	-0.761***	-0.317	1.12	3.318
	0.126	0.261	1.68	5.399
Missing DG	-0.507	-0.175	1.365	3.521
	0.479	0.512	1.757	5.431
Facility Effects	No	Yes	Yes	Yes
Patient Residence FE	Yes	Yes	Yes	Yes
Year FE	Yes	Yes	Yes	Yes
N	24160	24160	24160	24160
r2	0.464	0.473	0.467	0.48

* $p<0.10$, ** $p<0.05$, *** $p<0.01$. All standard errors were bootstrapped, stratifying by facility. The model was estimated without a constant, and there was no excluded disease category. The excluded racial category is all races other than white or black. Patient residence FE are fixed effects for all patient zipcodes associated with at least 150 patients. To account for any remaining variation, I also include a complete set of patient county fixed effects.

Table 7: Descriptive Statistics for Quality Estimates

	Obs	Mean	SD
D-FE	97	0.00	0.04
S-FE	97	0.00	0.17
E-FE	97	0.00	0.23
D-IV	73	0.01	0.23
S-IV	73	-0.01	0.64
E-IV	73	0.14	1.30
D-CF	97	-0.28	0.54
S-CF	97	-0.37	2.52
E-CF	97	0.20	2.82

Table 8: Correlation Matrix for Quality Estimates

	D-FE	D-IV	D-CF	E-FE	E-IV	E-CF	S-FE	S-IV	S-CF
D-FE	1.00								
D-IV	0.11	1.00							
D-CF	0.15	0.13	1.00						
E-FE	0.32	0.03	0.20	1.00					
E-IV	0.24	0.38	0.01	0.28	1.00				
E-CF	0.12	0.05	0.56	0.24	0.39	1.00			
S-FE	0.43	0.03	0.11	0.76	0.25	0.13	1.00		
S-IV	0.26	0.24	0.13	0.40	0.75	0.43	0.51	1.00	
S-CF	0.14	-0.08	0.71	0.28	0.21	0.82	0.16	0.36	1.00

D represents mortality models, S represents days in the ICU/CCU, and E represents days in the hospital.

Table 9: Decomposition of Facility Quality on Market and Facility Characteristics: CF Estimates

	Mortality b/se	Days in ICU/CCU b/se	Days Hospitalized b/se
Log(Total)	0.234**	1.096**	0.965**
	0.074	0.366	0.367
Share Affiliated	1.035**	4.118**	3.119*
	0.396	1.833	1.802
Facility Age	-0.001	0.012	0.012
	0.007	0.028	0.034
Non-Profit	0.163	0.939	1.071
	0.323	1.398	1.776
Alternative Large Firm	0.116	0.056	0.091
	0.135	0.58	0.723
Other	0.184	1.148+	0.8
	0.149	0.7	0.751
Constant	-1.299**	-5.076**	-3.726**
	0.304	1.435	1.392
N	97	97	97
r2	0.12	0.153	0.103

* $p<0.10$, ** $p<0.05$, *** $p<0.01$, + $p< 0.10$ in one-sided test. Standard errors bootstrapped with 500 replications.

Table 10: Decomposition of Facility Quality on Market and Facility Characteristics: FE and IV Estimates

	Mortality		Days in ICU/CCU		Days Hospitalized	
	FE	**IV**	**FE**	**IV**	**FE**	**IV**
	b/se	**b/se**	**b/se**	**b/se**	**b/se**	**b/se**
Log(Total)	0.001	-0.011	-0.028	0.011	0.027	0.037
	0.007	0.035	0.024	0.11	0.03	0.178
Share Affiliated	0.015	0.299*	-0.05	0.475	0.209	1.361*
	0.032	0.155	0.126	0.463	0.204	0.804
Facility Age	0	0.004	-0.001	-0.009	-0.006**	-0.014
	0	0.003	0.002	0.008	0.003	0.016
Non-Profit	-0.015	-0.112	-0.046	-0.089	-0.103	-0.712
	0.015	0.182	0.079	0.568	0.106	1.16
Alternative Large Firm	-0.004	-0.039	-0.011	-0.071	-0.031	0.079
	0.011	0.058	0.042	0.144	0.064	0.309
Other	0.017	0.064	0.049	0.145	0.116*	0.942**
	0.015	0.072	0.052	0.213	0.067	0.369
Constant	-0.015	-0.134	0.076	-0.15	-0.093	-0.666
	0.033	0.139	0.103	0.43	0.141	0.755
N	97	73	97	73	97	73
r2	0.046	0.112	0.058	0.047	0.126	0.124

* $p<0.10$, ** $p<0.05$, *** $p<0.01$, + $p< 0.10$ in one-sided test. Standard errors bootstrapped with 500 replications.

A Dataset Construction

Facility Data

I follow the same data cleaning procedures as in Wilson (2013). As described in that paper, the US-RDS data on yearly facility characteristics and activities are contained in the FACILITY dataset. Examining the connection between profit-status and chain affiliation in these data, it became evident that the raw USRDS data contained errors. In reality, all of the chains are universally either for- or non-profit. However, a non-trivial number of observations assign the "wrong" profit status to a facility affiliated with a given chain. Upon investigation, I came to the conclusion that much of the problem stemmed from lags in updating a given facility's status following a change in ownership. As a result, I imposed that a facility's for-profit status should match its chain affiliation.

The USRDS (2011) also warn that when a facility changes hands its identification number may also change. Thus, a facility would be seen to exit that did was not really liquidated, while another facility would appear to enter, though it would in truth be using old equipment and staff. Exploration of the data indicates that such events are uncommon insofar as most facilities known to be acquired remain in the data.

More commonly, I found that the data were sometimes slow to account for mergers. I addressed this problem by relying on the merger history provided in Cutler et al. (2012), imposing that facilities' affiliation should reflect whichever chain owned it for the bulk of the calendar year. In the econometric analyses, any noise introduced by erroneous cleaning should make it more difficult to cleanly identify differences across for- and non-profit facilities, and hence is a conservative approach.

Patient Data

The USRDS' patient-level data is spread across multiple different files, each focusing on different elements of potential interest. I constructed the data used in this paper as follows.

Patients' treatment history data – which are contained in RXHIST60 – are stratified by treatment modality and treating facility. Each distinct spell has a start and stop date. I merged these data with patients' time varying residence information – which is contained in RESIDENC – after limiting the residential information to places in Georgia. I further limited the data to individuals who moved more than three times within a given treatment regime. The concern is that such moves might indicate that the person was suffering from something unobservable that might make them an unrepresentative subject. This affected few patients. Subsequently, I merged the patient-treatment spell-residence information to the facility-year data. I then dropped all observations corresponding to treatment modalities other than hemodialysis received in facilitlies. I also excluded those individuals who shifted facilities within a year. Again, the concern is that the shift could be correlated with something outside of treatment, which it would be inappropriate to allow to be linked to the quality of treatment provided by either facility.

I subsequently merged in information on comorbidities – found in the MEDEVID dataset – and patient demographics – found in PATIENTS. From this information, I constructed a yearly measure of age by subtracting patients' birthyear from the current year.

Facilities – and the patients associated with them – were dropped if they did not perform 520 hemodialysis treatments in a year. I also focused only on those patients living in the zipcodes associated with the counties in the MSA according to the U.S. Census' Population Division.

Distance Data

Distances between places were constructed by the "Great Circle" method using the latitude and longitude centrums associated with zipcodes. The primary source of this information was the U.S. Census' ZCTA5 dataset. As zipcodes do not map perfectly to ZCTAs, some zipcodes in the data were not present in the ZCTA dataset. I used the information available at `brainyzip.com` to fill in these missing values.

Sample Construction

I initially mapped all of the facilities within the Atlanta MSA to all of the patients. Then as discussed in the text, I dropped the smaller of the set of observations further away than the chosen facility or the set of facilities further than 15 miles from the patients' zipcode of residence. I also dropped facilities that were not chosen in a given year at least 10 times as well as those that were not chosen at least 50 times overall. Eyeball checks indicate that – consistent with intuition – these facilities were in rural areas on the very outskirts of the Atlanta MSA.

Further details are available upon request.

B   Additional Tables

Table B-1: Choice Model Estimates

	b/se
Distance	-0.449***
	0.012
Distance^2	0.022***
	0
Distance*Years Treated	0.003***
	0
Distance*Age	-0.001***
	0
Distance*(Hypertension DG)	0.010**
	0.004
Distance*(Other Causes)	-0.001
	0.004
Distance*1(Black)	0
	0.008
Distance*1(White)	-0.007
	0.009
N	689265

* p<0.10, ** p<0.05, *** p<0.01.

Table B-2: Descriptive Statistics for Decomposition Variables

	Obs	Mean	SD
Nearby Facilities	98	14.83	12.73
Nearby Same Owner	98	3.46	4.50
Nearby Different Owner	98	11.37	10.17
Facility Age	98	10.87	8.28
County Population > 60	98	66049.30	42114.32
Number of Patients	98	246.53	305.02

Table B-3: Results for Model without Controls for Ownership

	Mortality CF b/se	Days in ICU/CCU CF b/se	Days Hospitalized CF b/se
Log(Total)	0.084*	0.443**	0.655**
	0.042	0.238	0.283
Facility Age	-0.002	0.009	-0.024
	0.004	0.021	0.027
Non-Profit	0.012	-0.416	-0.146
	0.182	0.994	1.228
Alternative Large Firm	0.139+	-0.194	-0.054
	0.095	0.519	0.651
Other	0.018	0.254	0.054
	0.1	0.518	0.634
Constant	-0.578**	-2.119**	-1.498**
	0.124	0.554	0.697
N	97	97	97
r2	0.037	0.056	0.073

* $p<0.10$, ** $p<0.05$, *** $p<0.01$, + $p< 0.10$ in one-sided test. Standard errors robust to heteroskedasticity. Observations weighted by number of patients.

Table B-4: Robustness Results: Weighting by Patients and Different Geographic Market Definition

	8 Mile Radius			Patient Weights		
	Mortality CF b/se	ICU/CCU CF b/se	Hosp. CF b/se	Mortality CF b/se	ICU/CCU CF b/se	Hosp. CF b/se
Log(Total)	0.262**	1.224**	1.073**	0.120**	0.801**	1.024**
	0.08	0.385	0.393	0.054	0.33	0.341
Share Affiliated	0.901**	3.646**	2.472+	0.391+	2.801**	2.725*
	0.373	1.757	1.771	0.258	1.403	1.473
Facility Age	-0.002	0.007	0.008	-0.003	0.005	-0.028
	0.007	0.028	0.034	0.005	0.021	0.027
Non-Profit	0.117	0.747	0.863	0.032	-0.272	-0.005
	0.322	1.39	1.775	0.179	0.972	1.204
Alternative Large Firm	0.149	0.198	0.221	0.161*	-0.037	0.098
	0.135	0.582	0.722	0.095	0.47	0.609
Other	0.161	1.077*	0.709	0.11	0.914*	0.697
	0.142	0.651	0.72	0.11	0.485	0.578
Constant	-1.252**	-4.912**	-3.453**	-0.860**	-4.137**	-3.462**
	0.292	1.363	1.319	0.215	1.088	1.093
N	97	97	97	97	97	97
r2	0.133	0.17	0.116	0.051	0.082	0.091

* $p<0.10$, ** $p<0.05$, *** $p<0.01$, + $p<0.10$ in one-sided test. Standard errors robust to heteroskedasticity. Observations weighted by number of patients.

Table B-5: Robustness Result: Per Capita Market Structure

	Centers per Capita		
	Mortality CF b/se	Days in ICU/CCU CF b/se	Days Hospitalized CF b/se
Affiliated per 1000	0.283+	1.338+	0.739
	0.189	0.833	0.799
Other per 1000	-0.018	-0.032	0.001
	0.072	0.326	0.378
Facility Age	0	0.019	0.022
	0.007	0.029	0.035
Non-Profit	0.274	1.5	1.553
	0.345	1.441	1.916
Alternative Large Firm	0.104	0.002	-0.154
	0.147	0.609	0.736
Other	0.102	0.888	0.38
	0.175	0.778	0.802
Constant	-0.471**	-1.617**	-0.62
	0.16	0.657	0.707
N	97	97	97
r2	0.054	0.095	0.052

* p<0.10, ** p<0.05, *** p<0.01, + p< 0.10 in one-sided test. Standard errors robust to heteroskedasticity. Observations weighted by number of patients.